Slow Cooker Cookbook

Delicious Slow Cooker Recipes for the Crockpot

Kathleen Lee

Copyright © 2013 Kathleen Lee
All rights reserved.

Table of Contents

INTRODUCTION **1**
    What Is The Difference Between a Slow Cooker and a Crock Pot? 1
    Slow Cookers and Food Safety 3
    The Advantages to Cooking with a Slow Cooker 3
    Tips For Making The Most Of Your Slow Cooker 4
    You Can Even Make Meatloaf In the Slow Cooker! 6

BREAKFAST RECIPES **8**
    Cranberry Oatmeal 8
    Raspberry Coconut Rice Pudding 10
    Turkey Bacon and Egg Casserole 12
    Breakfast Cheese Strata with Vegetables 14
    Cherry Croissant Pudding 17
    Hash Brown Casserole 19

SNACK, DESSERT, AND APPETIZER RECIPES **21**
    Quick Chocolate Nut Clusters 21
    Quick Tapioca Pudding 23
    Hummus 25
    Chocolate Mocha Bread Pudding 27
    Carrot Cake 29
    Peach Cheesecake 30

SOUP AND STEW RECIPES **32**
    Chunky Chicken Stew 32
    Italian Turkey Sausage Stew 34
    Chicken Noodle Cream Soup 36
    Turkey Stew 37
    French Onion Soup 40
    Split Pea Soup 41
    Mexican Tortilla Soup 42

MAIN DISH AND ONE DISH MEALS **44**
    Famous Beef Pot Roast 44

Corned Beef Brisket and Cabbage 46
Mexican Chicken Fajita Casserole 48
Spicy Beef Pot Roast and Noodles 50
Macaroni and Cheese Crock 53
Black Bean Chili 55
Beefy Noodles 57
Shredded Turkey Sandwiches 59
Round Steak 61
Shrimp Creole Casserole 63
Jamaica Chicken 65
Jambalaya 67
Spicy Black-Eyed Peas 69
Beef Pepper Steak 71
Vegetarian Chili 73
Chicken and Dumplings 75
French Dip Au Jus 77
Chicken Stroganoff 79
Spaghetti 80

5 DAY MEAL PLAN 82

CONCLUSION 85

Introduction

What Is The Difference Between a Slow Cooker and a Crock Pot?

The old style cookers were called "slow cookers," where the heating element is in a separate unit from the main food holder. Actually, larger slow cookers and "crock pots" still come this way. When the "crock pot" made the scene, it was with the heating element cased within the food holder all in one. If you were lucky you had a removable plug for easy cleaning. Not so lucky were the ones where the plug was a permanent fixture. Crock Pot, by the way, is a registered trademark by the Rival Manufacturing Company, but their name brand became a nickname for slow cookers.

Some slow cookers may have the heating elements that surround the food holder, helping to give it even heat. Others may only have the heating element on the bottom, causing the need for extra stirring to keep from burning and sticking with the food.

Slow cookers come in three sizes, with a 3.5, 4 and 5 quarts being the most popular sizes. Obviously if a recipe serves 12 you will not want to try to cook it in a 3.5 quart sized slow cooker. Most people only have one or two sizes and know how to adjust. Normally, if you have a larger family, you will have a larger slow cooker. It helps to eyeball the food. You want the slow cooker to be filled to at least half way point, but you do not want it bubbling over the top. So consider the size of the foods you are going to cook and gauge whether or not you need a small or large slow cooker. Most of the recipes here do well with a 4 to 5 quart slow cooker.

When purchasing a slow cooker you need to decide first how big of one you need. Obviously if you are cooking for only two or three people, you would do well with a smaller one. If you have a large family, you need a smaller one. Also, consider whether or not you wish to cook extra to freeze and eat later or to have meals for a couple of days. People are finding this an excellent way to save on groceries and energy, to cook a double or triple portion and eat on it for a few days.

When you purchase a new slow cooker be sure to read all the instructions. It will help save you time in the long run and will help to preserve the unit.

Slow Cookers and Food Safety

Some may wonder if when cooking a meal for 8 hours on a low setting, if the food is safe, or will bacteria grow. It is a legitimate concern, but needless for a slow cooker that is in good shape. Most all slow cookers are set for their lowest temperatures to be above 140 degrees Fahrenheit, the temperature that most bacteria are killed. It helps if you are cooking beef, to brown it ahead of time. That way when you put it into the slow cooker it will already be hot. You do not want the slow cooker getting so hot it easily burns the food. If that were the case, you would not want to go to sleep or leave for the day with the slow cooker cooking. If the temperature of the meat is a concern, you can always stick a meat thermometer into it to test it prior to eating.

The Advantages to Cooking with a Slow Cooker

Foods often bloom with flavor if they are allowed to cook slowly, allowing the different flavors to melt together. You know how good some leftovers taste? Well cooking in a slow cooker is like having fresh foods with that have the flavors distributed perfectly.

Because slow cookers are not so hot to burn, you are

less likely to have burned meals. This makes everyone happy.

Even the most inexpensive cuts of meat, which would normally be too tough to eat, will fall off the fork and melt in the mouth after 4 to 8 hours of cooking in a slow cooker.

It saves energy to cook with a slow cooker because, in most cases, you will not have to run an oven for a lengthy time. Running an oven to cook something like a pot roast can take several hours and uses a lot more electricity or gas. The slow cooker runs on a normal outlet and uses less electricity. Some recipes do call for a bit of extra cooking for preparation of the full meal.

One dish meals are easy to cook and easy to clean up. There is no worry with many pots and pans, with having to scrub the stove and oven after a meal. Just clean the slow cooker and you are done.

Tips For Making The Most Of Your Slow Cooker

When shopping for the ingredients in the recipes here and for any foods you plan to put in the slow cooker, consider the size of the slow cooker you have compared to the size of the food you need. If a recipe calls for a roast, try to find one in the shape that will easily fit down in the slow cooker. Many times you can either cut it up to fit, or trim the fat to make more room.

When cooking root vegetables you should lay them in the slow cooker first, under the meat (unless the directions say otherwise). This helps the root vegetables to tenderize better and cook faster.

When cooking a meal it helps to taste test first, to make sure you've added enough seasonings. While it's still bubbly and hot is the best time to add more seasonings if necessarily. Some people even recommend to wait until the last hour or half hour to add the seasonings, so they will burst right when you are ready to eat. The other argument about adding them in the beginning is to help the flavor to disperse throughout the dish. This is where you need to test the theories and determine which way to go. Some meals may be best to wait to season at the end, while others may be best to season at the beginning.

When foods cook, especially slowly, they tend to lose their coloring. You may have noticed this when cooking stews in the slow cooker. You can help make it vibrant again by garnishing with colorful foods at the end, such as tossing in some green scallions, chives, tomatoes, etc. Use your judgment for an added garnishment to add color and a pop of flavor. Not all dishes need this.

When cooking dried beans it is always best to soak them the night before cooking in the slow cooker. If you do not do this, they may be tough and not tenderize right.

Aside from the recipes below, you can cook just about anything in a slow cooker. Dairy-based ingredients tend to burn and stick, so go easy on those. But you can take a cheap cut of meat and put it in the slow cooker and pour broth over it and cook it on low for 8 hours and have a meat dish that is tender and tasty. You can fill it with the ingredients for cheese dip (with often stirring) and allow it to make the dip during a couple of hours. Or fill it with ingredients for hot cocoa and be able to serve a crowd with ease.

You Can Even Make Meatloaf In the Slow Cooker!

You can even cook a meatloaf in the slow cooker. There is not a recipe for this below, so we will share it here. Just make the meatloaf recipe the way you normally do. Take enough aluminum foil out and fold it lengthwise to sit within the slow cooker with enough over the top, to be the handles. You will want to use at least two or three of these, and lay them down so the meatloaf sits on them. Fold them into one-inch wide strips. Mold the meatloaf to fit nicely within the slow cooker. Try to make it where the sides are not touching, but if they do that is okay. Place the meatloaf on the foil strips and cover it. Cook for 8 hours on low, or 4 to 5 on high. You may want to test the temperature in the center with a meat thermometer to make sure it is hot enough. This enables you to cook the meatloaf and not have to be there to watch it like you would in the oven.

Breakfast Recipes

Cranberry Oatmeal

Nothing quite satisfies a tummy like a nice hot bowl of oatmeal first thing in the morning. Often people do not make it because of a time factor. We have taken care of that by putting it into a slow cooker to cook all night and be nice and hot for breakfast.

What You'll Need:

4 cups of water
2 cups of cranberries (dried)
1 cup of oats (steel cut works best)
1/2 cup of cream (half-and-half)
4 teaspoons of brown sugar
4 pats of butter

How to Make It:

Place the 4 cups of water into a slow cooker and stir in the cup of steel cut oats followed by the 2 cups of dried cranberries. Stir in the 1/2 cup of half-and-half cream and the 4 teaspoons of brown sugar. Cook on low over

night (8 hours). Stir prior to dividing into 4 bowls. Add a pat of butter and stir. Enjoy.
Makes 4 servings.

Raspberry Coconut Rice Pudding

Sometimes a nice hot bowl of rice pudding just hits the spot in the morning. This pudding is rich and creamy and everyone loves it. It makes a great snack too.

What You'll Need:

3 cups of coconut water
1 1/2 cups of coconut milk
1 1/2 cups of water
1 1/4 cups of rice (short grain brown)
1/2 cup of sugar (granulated)
2 tablespoons of butter
1 tablespoon of vanilla extract
1 teaspoon of lime zest
raspberries (as needed)

How to Make It:

Spray the slow cooker with cooking spray to prevent sticking. Add the 3 cups of coconut water, 1 1/2 cups of coconut milk 1 1/2 cups of water, 1/2 cup of granulated sugar, and the tablespoon of vanilla extract and stir. Add the 1 1/4 cups of short grain brown rice and stir one more time. Turn the slow cooker to high and cover and cook for about 5 and a half hours (or get up and turn on the slow cooker about that much time prior to breakfast). In the morning, turn the slow cooker off and uncover and stir. Let sit for 15 minutes. Pour into a large serving bowl, add the 2 tablespoons of butter and the teaspoon of lime zest, and stir. Serve and top with raspberries as desired.

Makes 10-12 servings.

Turkey Bacon and Egg Casserole

Imagine waking up to the smell of bacon and eggs first thing in the morning and the kitchen will be clean too. This delicious recipe will have the house smelling of favorite breakfast foods. Serve with toast or biscuits.

What You'll Need:

1 pound of turkey bacon
1 dozen eggs
4 cups of hash browns (frozen)
1 1/2 cups of cheddar cheese (sharp - shredded)
1 cup of milk
1/2 cup of onion (chopped)
1/2 cup of bell pepper (green chopped)
1 tablespoon of olive oil
salt and pepper to taste

How to Make It:

First, insure no sticking by spraying the slow cooker with cooking spray.
Prep: Add the tablespoon of olive oil to a skillet and heat to medium. Sauté the 1/2 cups of chopped onions and green bell peppers. Set aside for a few minutes to cool.

Next, layer the ingredients inside the slow cooker. Place 1 1/3 cup of the frozen hash browns into the bottom of the slow cooker. Cut the turkey bacon into bite-sized chunks and layer 1/3 of the package on top of the hash browns along with a third of the sautéed peppers and onions and the shredded sharp cheddar cheese. Do this twice again.

Crack the dozen eggs into a large mixing bowl and add the cup of milk and salt and pepper. Whisk until smooth and pour into the slow cooker over the top of the hash brown, peppers and onions, turkey bacon and cheddar cheese. Cover the slow cooker and cook overnight, for around 8 hours. Alternatively, if you wish to make this for a supper, it can cook in 5 hours on high.

Makes 10-12 servings.

Breakfast Cheese Strata with Vegetables

This breakfast casserole will satisfy and give energy with the savory mix of vegetables, herbs, and spices. Try it for lunch or supper too.

What You'll Need:

1 dozen eggs
1 pound loaf of sourdough bread (no crust, cut into bite-sized cubes)
2 cups of cheddar cheese (extra sharp shredded)
1 1/2 cups of milk
1 cup of tomatoes (plum, cut lengthwise, seeds removed)
1 cup of turkey ham (diced)
1/2 cup of heavy cream
1 tablespoon of butter (+1 teaspoon)
1 tablespoon of parsley (minced flat leaf)
1 1/2 teaspoons of chives (dried)
1 teaspoon of salt (+ dashes divided)
1/4 teaspoon of black pepper
1/8 teaspoon of nutmeg (ground)
1/8 teaspoon of cayenne pepper

How to Make It:

Make ahead 2 days before - First, preheat the oven to 250 degrees Fahrenheit. place the tomatoes, meat side up, on a baking sheet in the oven in a single layer, sprinkle with salt. Bake for 5 1/2 hours. Store in a container in the refrigerator.

The day before - After the tomatoes are ready, spray a slow cooker with cooking spray. Add the eggs to a large bowl and beat, mix in the 1 1/2 cups of milk, 1/2 cup of heavy cream, teaspoon of salt, 1/4 teaspoon of black pepper, 1/8 teaspoon of ground nutmeg, and the 1/8 teaspoon of cayenne pepper. In a separate bowl add the cup of oven baked plum tomatoes, cup of diced turkey ham, tablespoon of minced flat leaf parsley, and the 1 1/2 teaspoons of dried chives and toss to combine.

Sprinkle 1 cup of the sharp cheddar cheese on the bottom of the slow cooker. Next add one-third of the pound of bread cubes, next add half of the tomato mixture. Add another one third of the bread cubes, then the remaining half of the tomato mixture. Finally top with the remaining one-third of the bread cubes and the remaining cup of extra sharp cheddar cheese. Pour the egg batter over the food in the slow cooker, making sure all parts are moist from the eggs. Melt the tablespoon plus teaspoon of butter and drizzle it over the top of the food. Set the entire covered container in the refrigerator for 8 hours or overnight. Next day, cook on high for 4 hours or low for 8 hours.

Makes 8 servings.

Cherry Croissant Pudding

This is a different twist with the famed croissant and with delicious bread pudding. Makes for a tasty breakfast or even a delicious dessert.

What You'll Need:

8 croissants (ripped into thirds)
3 cups of milk
1 cup of light cream
2/3 cup of cherries (dried)
1/3 cup of apple juice
1/3 cup of brown sugar
4 eggs (beaten)
2 teaspoons of vanilla extract
dash of salt

How to Make It:

Add the 2/3 cup of dried cherries to a microwave safe bowl and stir in the 1/3 cup of apple juice. Microwave on high for 60 seconds. Set aside for 15 minutes. In a separate large bowl, combine the 3 cups of milk with the cup of light cream, 1/3 cup of brown sugar, 4 beaten eggs, 2 teaspoons of vanilla extract, and the dash of salt. Spray the slow cooker bottom with cooking spray. Place

1/3 of the ripped croissants in the bottom of the slow cooker. Pour 1/3 of the egg batter over the croissants, place 1/3 of the cherry mixture. Repeat the layers twice again. Pour any remaining liquid from the cherries over the top. Refrigerate for 4 hours. Then cook on low for 8 hours. Garnish with your favorite syrup if desired when serving.

Makes 8 servings.

Hash Brown Casserole

This is always a favorite, the delicious flavor of turkey bacon and turkey sausage combined with the cheese and hash browns makes the mouth water for more.

What You'll Need:

6 slices of turkey bacon
6 cups of hash browns (frozen)
1 1/2 cups of turkey sausage
1/2 cup of onion (chopped)
1/2 cup of bell pepper (red chopped)
1/2 cup of Colby cheese (shredded)
1/2 cup of Monterey Jack cheese (shredded)
1 jar of cheddar cheese pasta sauce (16 oz.)
1 can of mushrooms (sliced and drained 4 oz.)
canola oil

How to Make It:

First, cook the 6 slices of turkey bacon in a little canola oil in the skillet, cool and crumble into pieces. Next cook the turkey sausage, adding more canola oil if needed. Add the 1/2 cup of chopped onions to the sausage while it is cooking. Make sure the sausage is well crumbled.

Spray the bottom of the slow cooker with cooking spray, and place in this order the cooked bacon, cooked sausage and onions, 6 cups of frozen hash browns, 1/2 cups of shredded Colby and Monterey Jack cheeses, can of drained mushrooms, then the 1/2 cup of chopped red bell pepper. With a large spoon, stir and toss the food. Last, pour the jar of cheddar cheese pasta sauce. Cover and cook for 8 hours on low.

Makes 6 servings.

Snack, Dessert, and Appetizer Recipes

Quick Chocolate Nut Clusters

This recipe is "quick" because it only takes 3 hours in the slow cooker. This recipe calls for walnuts, but you can substitute pecans or peanuts if you wish.

What You'll Need:

7 cups of walnuts (chopped)
20 squares of almond bark
4 squares of sweet chocolate squares (baking chocolate)
2 cups of chocolate chips (semisweet)

How to Make It:

Prep: Set out 36 cupcake liners on a tray.

Place the 7 cups of chopped nuts into the bottom of the slow cooker. Place the 4 squares of sweet chocolate over the nuts. Sprinkle the 2 cups of semisweet chocolate chips over the sweet chocolate squares and nuts. Layer the 20 squares of almond bark on top. Place a lid on the slow cooker and turn to low, cooking for 3 hours. After the three hours, stir with a warmed metal spoon or use a wooden or plastic spoon. Evenly spoon the chocolate nut mixture into the 36 cupcake liners. Set aside and allow to cool and harden. Enjoy. (It is okay to set in the refrigerator to cool faster.)

Quick Tapioca Pudding

A delicious favorite, tapioca pudding made "fast" in the slow cooker, taking just 2 hours from prep to finish.

What You'll Need:

2 1/2 cups of milk
2 cups of water (cold)
1/2 cup of tapioca (large pearl)
1/2 cup of cream (heavy)
1/3 cup of sugar (granulated)
1 egg yolk
3 teaspoons of lemon zest
salt

How to Make It:

Prep: Place the 1/2 cup of large pearl tapioca in a bowl and add the 2 cups of cold water. Cover the bowl and set aside for 8 hours or overnight. After the soak, strain out the water and place the pearls into the slow cooker. Turn to high and add the 2 1/2 cups of milk, 1/2 cup of heavy cream and a dash or two of salt. Cover and cook for about 2 hours. Stir often.

Add the egg yolk and the 1/3 cup of granulated sugar to

a bowl and mix with a whisk. Pull out 1 cup of the hot tapioca mixture; allow it to cool for a few minutes. Add a spoonful at a time to the egg batter, slowly to allow the eggs to temper and not cook. Stir well. Gradually add the egg mixture into the slow cooker, stirring to mix. Stir in the 3 teaspoons of lemon zest. Cover and cook for another 15 minutes, stirring every 5 minutes. Pour the pudding into a large serving bowl and cover with plastic wrap to keep a skin from forming. Set aside for at least 60 minutes before placing in the refrigerator. Serve chilled.

Hummus

Hummus goes well with pita chips and makes a great healthy appetizer.

What You'll Need:

1 pound of chickpeas (dried, sorted, rinsed)
7 1/4 cups of water (divided)
1/3 cup of lemon juice
1/3 cup of tahini
1/4 cup of olive oil (extra virgin)
1 1/2 teaspoons of salt
1 teaspoon of garlic (minced)
1/4 teaspoon of baking soda

How to Make It:

First, place the pound of dried, sorted and rinsed chickpeas into a slow cooker, pour the 7 cups of water over the top and stir in the 1/4 teaspoon of baking soda. Cover the peas and cook on low overnight (for 8 1/2 hours) or cook on high for 4 hours. Turn off and cool for a few minutes, then pour into a strainer to drain the water. Pour the drained peas into a food processor or blender along with the 1 1/2 teaspoons of salt and the teaspoon of minced garlic. Turn on and process for just under half a minute. Stop to stir and combine, scraping the sides. Pour in the 1/3 cup of tahini and process for another half a minute. Stop to stir and scrape. Turn back on and slowly add the 1/4 cup of extra virgin olive oil and the 1/3 cup of lemon juice. Put the hummus into a serving bowl and enjoy with chips or crackers.

Chocolate Mocha Bread Pudding

The steamy decadent bowl of chocolate bread pudding will bring your senses alive as you spoon in a mouth full of this delicious dessert.

What You'll Need:

1 pound of French bread (cubed)
8 oz. of chocolate (semisweet grated)
6 eggs (lightly beaten)
3 cups of milk
1 cup of sugar (granulated)
1 cup of brown sugar (light and packed)
1/2 cup of coffee (strong and black)
1/4 cup of cocoa powder
1/4 cup of heavy cream
1 tablespoon of vanilla extract
2 teaspoons of almond extract
1 1/2 teaspoons of cinnamon (ground)
Whipped cream for garnishment

How to Make It:

Spray the bottom of the slow cooker with cooking spray. Layer the cubed French bread on the bottom. In a large bowl add the 3 cups of milk with the 1/2 cup of strong black coffee, and the 1/4 cup of heavy cream and stir with a whisk. In a separate bowl, add the cup of granulate sugar, cup of light brown sugar, with the 1/4 cup of cocoa powder and mix. Gradually add the sugars and cocoa into the milk mixture. In yet another bowl, stir together the 1 tablespoon of vanilla extract and the 2 teaspoons of almond extract and add to the 6 lightly beaten eggs. Stir in the 1 1/2 teaspoons of ground cinnamon. Add the egg mixture to the milk mixture and stir. Stir in the 8 ounces of grated semisweet chocolate. Pour the batter over the cubed bread in the slow cooker. Let it sit for about 20 minutes before turning on the slow cooker. Turn on the cooker on low for 8 hours or high for 4 hours. Check the middle of the pudding by inserting a knife. Pudding is done if the knife comes out clean, if it does not; continue to cook it until it does. Serve in a bowl, top with whipped cream.

Carrot Cake

Here is a delicious carrot cake made from the slow cooker and best topped with whipped topping.

What You'll Need:

1 box of cake mix (spice cake 18.25 oz.)
1 box of pudding mix (butterscotch, instant)
2 cups of carrots (finely shredded)
1 cup of water
1 cup of pineapples (crushed)
1 cup of sour cream
4 eggs (beaten)
whipped topping (garnishment)

How to Make It:
Spray the bottom of the slow cooker with cooking spray. Mix the 1 box of cake mix, 1 box of butterscotch instant pudding mix, 2 cups of carrots (finely shredded), 1 cup of water, 1 cup of pineapples (crushed), 1 cup of sour cream with the 4 eggs using an electric mixer for 2 minutes on medium. Pour into the slow cooker. Place the lid on and cook on low for 5 hours. Serve warm with a dollop of whipped topping.

Makes 10 servings.

Peach Cheesecake

A decadent cheesecake complete with a graham cracker pie crust.

What You'll Need:

1 container of ricotta cheese (15 ounce)
1 graham cracker pie crust (9 inch)
1 can of peaches (chopped 15 oz.)
3/4 cup of sugar (granulated + 1 tablespoon)
1/3 cup of orange juice
3 eggs
2 tablespoons of orange zest
2 teaspoons of cornstarch
1 teaspoon of vanilla extract
pinches of salt

How to Make It:

This is a 2 part cooking, first in slow cooker, 2nd in oven. First, run the container of ricotta cheese through the food processor or blender to make it smooth. Scrape the sides, but add to it the 3/4 cup of granulated sugar and turn to puree for 60 seconds. Scrape the sides, add the 3 eggs, 2 tablespoons of orange zest and the teaspoon of vanilla extract along with the pinch of salt. Puree until combined and silky smooth (like cheesecake). Pour into the graham cracker pie crust. Place an oven safe small bowl in the bottom of the slow cooker. Set the cheesecake on top, if it is not secure, set an oven safe plate on the bowl, then set the cheesecake on it. Cover and cook on high for 90 minutes. Remove cheesecake from slow cooker to cool for half an hour, then refrigerate for another half an hour. Meanwhile place a saucepan on the stove. Pour in the peach juice from the can of peaches along with the tablespoon of granulated sugar, 1/3 cup of orange juice, 2 teaspoons of cornstarch, and a pinch of salt. With the heat on medium, stir and add the peaches from the can. Stir and cook for 5 minutes. Pour over the cheesecake. Serve and enjoy.

Makes 6 to 8 servings.

Soup and Stew Recipes

Chunky Chicken Stew

Nothing is quite as hearty or comforting as a delicious chunky soup made of lean chicken breasts and chocked full of healthy vegetables.

What You'll Need:

2 chicken breasts
1 can of navy beans (15 oz., drained and rinsed)
1 can of tomatoes (undrained stewed - 14.5 oz.)
3 1/2 cups of chicken broth
2 cups of carrots (chopped)
2 cups of cabbage (finely shredded)
1 cup of peas (frozen green)
1/2 cup of onion (diced)
1/2 teaspoon of salt (divided)
1/2 teaspoon of pepper (divided)
1/2 teaspoon of thyme (fresh finely chopped)
1 bay leaf

How to Make It:

Cut the 2 chicken breasts in half and sprinkle the 1/4 teaspoon of salt and 1/8 teaspoon of pepper all over. Place the seasoned chicken breast halves in the bottom of the slow cooker. Turn to low. Add the drained rinsed can of navy beans, can of stewed tomatoes (undrained), 3 1/2 cups of chicken broth, 2 cups of chopped carrots, 2 cups of shredded cabbage, 1 cup of frozen green peas, 1/2 cup of diced onion, 1/4 teaspoon of salt, remainder of the 1/2 teaspoon of pepper, 1/2 teaspoon of fresh finely chopped thyme, and the bay leaf. Cover and cook overnight for about 8 hours. (if you need it faster turn it to high and cook for 4 hours.)

After it has cooked, remove the bay leaf and the chicken breast halves. Discard the bay leaf. Shred the chicken breasts with a fork and replace the chicken to the soup. Salt and pepper to taste when serving.

Italian Turkey Sausage Stew

This hearty stew incorporates lean turkey sausage with beans to make a meal that will satisfy.

What You'll Need:

1 pound of Italian turkey sausage (cut into bite sized chunks)
1 can of tomatoes (14.5 ounce, fire-roasted diced, undrained)
3 cups of chicken broth
2 cups of onions (half inch strips)
1 cup of navy beans (dried, rinsed and sorted)
2/3 cup of carrots (chopped fine)
1/2 cup of Parmesan + more for garnish
1/2 cup of macaroni noodles
7 sprigs of thyme (keep together on stem)
2 tablespoons of parsley (fresh chopped)
2 teaspoons of vinegar (balsamic)
2 teaspoons of garlic (minced)
salt and pepper to taste

How to Make It:

First, add the2 cups of onions to the slow cooker followed by the 2 pounds of bite-sized Italian turkey sausage, cup of dried, rinsed, and sorted navy beans, 2/3 cup of finely chopped carrots, the 7 sprigs of thyme, and the 2 teaspoons of minced garlic. In a separate bowl add the can of fire-roasted diced tomatoes with the 3 cups of chicken broth and stir until mixed. Pour over the sausage and vegetables in the slow cooker. Sprinkle the 1/2 cup of Parmesan over the top. Place a cover over the slow cooker and turn to low for 8 hours (or cook on high for 4 hours). Once cooked, carefully remove the 7 thyme sprigs. Stir in the 1/2 cup of macaroni noodles, replace cover, and cook for another 20 minutes, until the pasta is tender. Transfer the stew to a large serving bowl. Sprinkle salt, pepper, and Parmesan cheese to taste. Delicious served with bread or rolls.

Makes 8 servings.

Chicken Noodle Cream Soup

This pot of soup is hearty and delicious using rotisserie chicken with a can of mushroom soup to make it creamy.

What You'll Need:

1 rotisserie chicken (the kind you buy, already cooked from the grocers deli section)
1 large can of cream of mushroom soup (condensed with roasted garlic)
7 cups of chicken broth
1 cup of onions (diced)
1 cup of celery (diced)
1 cup of carrots (diced)
1/2 cup of egg noodles (uncooked)
1/4 teaspoon of chervil
1/4 teaspoon of chives (dried)
1/4 teaspoon of parsley (dried)
1/4 teaspoon of tarragon
salt and pepper to taste

How to Make It:

First, shred the rotisserie chicken meat discarding the bones and skin. Place in the slow cooker. Add the cups of diced onions, celery, and carrots. Pour the 7 cups of chicken broth into a large bowl and add the large can of cream of mushroom soup. Stir using a whisk to smooth out the chunks. Pour the liquid over the chicken and vegetables and stir in the 1/4 teaspoon of chervil, 1/4 teaspoon of dried chives, 1/4 teaspoon of dried parsley, and the 1/4 teaspoon of tarragon. Salt and pepper while stirring. Cover the slow cooker and cook on high for 8 hours or on low for 4 hours. During the last 20 minutes of cook time add the 1/2 cup of uncooked egg noodles. Salt and pepper to taste and enjoy.

Makes 8 servings.

Turkey Stew

This turkey stew is chocked full of vegetables and fruits to make it a wonderfully filling and delightfully tasty meal.

What You'll Need:

4 turkey thigh (skinless)
2 cans of chickpeas (15.5 oz., drained, rinsed)
1 can of tomatoes (28 oz., chunked and peeled, undrained)

2 red chilies (whole dried)
4 cups of carrots (chunked)
2 cups of cilantro (fresh cut)
1 1/2 cups of onions (wedges)
1 cup of parsley (fresh cut)
1 cup of apricots (dried)
1/2 cup of olive oil (extra virgin)
1/2 cup of raisins (golden)
1/2 cup of butternut squash (chunks)
1 tablespoon of lemon juice
4 teaspoons of salt (divided)
1 teaspoon of allspice (ground)
1/2 teaspoon of garlic (minced)
1/2 teaspoon of cumin (ground)

How to Make It:

Put the 3 teaspoons of salt together with the teaspoon of ground allspice and mix. Take half of the seasoning and rub into the 4 turkey thighs. Place the seasoned turkey thighs in the slow cooker. Mix the remaining seasoning with the 2 cans of drained, rinsed, chickpeas, can of chunked peeled tomatoes, 2 red chilies, 4 cups of chunked carrots, 1 1/2 cups of onion wedges, cup of apricots, and the 1/2 cup of golden raisins and pour over the turkey legs in the slow cooker. Turn to high, cover, and cook for 6 hours or on low for 8 hours. After cooked, pull the turkey meat from the bones and discard the bones. Pour the vegetables into a large serving bowl. Place the turkey meat on top of the vegetables. Add the 2 cups of fresh cut cilantro, cup of fresh parsley, teaspoon of salt, 1/2 teaspoon of minced garlic, and the 1/2 teaspoon of ground cumin into a food processor. Process while drizzling in the 1/2 cup of extra virgin olive oil and the tablespoon of lemon juice. Serve the turkey stew in bowls, drizzle the parsley and cilantro sauce over the top, and enjoy.

Makes 4 servings.

French Onion Soup

A favorite for many, this soup goes great as part of a 4 or 5 course meal or as a delicious lunch.

What You'll Need:

1 loaf of French bread (cut into 8 slices)
3 1/2 cups of beef broth
2 1/2 cups of onions (sliced thin)
1 cup of Swiss cheese (shredded)
2 cans of beef consommé (10 oz. cans)
1 packet of onion soup mix

How to Make It:

Add the 3 1/2 cups of beef broth to the slow cooker along with the 2 1/2 cups of thin sliced onions, 2 cans of beef consommé and the packet of onion soup mix. Cover the slow cooker and cook on low for 8 hours or high for 4. When cooked, pour soup into a serving bowl. Place the 8 slices of French bread onto a baking sheet. Evenly disperse the cup of shredded Swiss cheese on the 8 slices of French bread and place under the broiler until the cheese melts. Ladle the soup into bowls, and place the hot cheesy French bread on top of the soup, or to the side if you prefer.

Split Pea Soup

Split pea soup makes the perfect comfort food on a cold day or a nice light meal on a summer day.

What You'll Need:

1 pound of green split peas
10 cups of chicken broth
1/2 pound of spicy turkey sausage
1 1/2 cups of carrots (diced)
1 cup of onions (diced)
1 cup of celery (diced)
2 bay leaves
1 teaspoon of garlic (minced)
salt and pepper

How to Make It:

Add the 1 pound of green split peas, 10 cups of chicken broth, 1/2 pound of spicy, turkey sausage, 1 1/2 cups of carrots (diced), 1 cup of onions (diced), 1 cup of celery (diced), 2 bay leaves and the 1 teaspoon of garlic (minced) to the slow cooker. Place a lid on and cook on low setting for 8 hours or high for 4 hours. Once cooked, remove the 2 bay leaves and add salt and pepper to taste. Delicious served with corn muffins.

Mexican Tortilla Soup

A satisfying bowl of soup is good for lunch or supper and hearty enough to be eaten alone.

What You'll Need:

1 pound of chicken breasts (boneless and skinless)
7 corn tortillas
1 can of tomatoes (whole and mashed 15 oz.)
1 can of enchilada sauce (10 oz.)
1 package of corn (frozen 10 oz.)
1 can of chili peppers (green 4 oz.)
1/2 cup of onion (chopped)
1 bay leaf
1 tablespoon of cilantro (chopped)
1 teaspoon of garlic (minced)
1 teaspoon of cumin (ground)
1 teaspoon of chili powder (ground)
1 teaspoon of salt
1/4 teaspoon of pepper (black)
canola oil
water
chicken broth

How to Make It:

Put the pound of chicken breasts in the bottom of the slow cooker along with the can of whole mashed tomatoes, can of enchilada sauce, can of green chili peppers, 1/2 cup of chopped onions and the teaspoon of minced garlic. In a bowl, add a cup of water and a cup of chicken broth and combine with the teaspoon of minced garlic, teaspoon of ground cumin, teaspoon of ground chili powder, teaspoon of salt, and the 1/4 teaspoon of black pepper. Pour over the chicken and add more equal amounts of water and chicken broth until completely covered. Stir in the package of frozen corn and the tablespoon of chopped cilantro. Cover with a lid and cook on low for 7 hours or on high for 3 1/2 hours. Remove the chicken and shred with a fork. Replace the chicken, but turn the slow cooker off. Preheat the oven to 400 degrees Fahrenheit. Brush some canola oil onto the tortillas and cut into "chip sized" strips. Bake on a baking sheet for about 12 minutes. Serve with the soup.

Makes 8 servings.

Main Dish and One Dish Meals

Famous Beef Pot Roast

There is nothing quite as special as the smell of a slow cooker of pot roast wafting through the house. Serve this up with a platter of steamed carrots and potatoes.

What You'll Need:

1 chuck roast (at least 3 pounds)
1 can of cream of mushroom soup (condensed 10.75 oz.)
1/2 cup of onions (sliced thin)
1/2 cup of white grape juice
1/4 cup of canola oil
4 beef bouillon cubes (crushed)
3 bay leaves
1 teaspoon of garlic (minced)
2/3 teaspoon of salt
1/3 teaspoon of pepper
1/3 teaspoon of garlic powder

How to Make It:

Rub the 2/3 teaspoon of salt, 1/3 teaspoon of pepper,

and the 1/3 teaspoon of garlic powder onto the raw 3 pound chuck roast. Heat a skillet to medium high. Add the 1/4 cup of canola oil. Brown the seasoned chuck roast. Place the browned seasoned chuck roast into the slow cooker. Add the 1/2 cup of thin sliced onions, 4 crushed beef bouillon cubes, 3 bay leaves, and the teaspoon of minced garlic. Pour the 1/2 cup of white grape juice over the top. Place a lid on the slow cooker and cook on low for eight hours. Remove and discard the 3 bay leaves and chunk up the pot roast prior to serving.

Corned Beef Brisket and Cabbage

This is a favorite Irish dish that can be enjoyed by anyone year round.

What You'll Need:

4 pounds of corned beef brisket (uncooked with seasoning packet)
1/2 head of cabbage (wedged)
4 1/2 cups of water (hot)
3 cups of rutabaga (cut into halves and wedges)
3 cups of potatoes (cut into bite size)
1 1/2 cups of carrots (chunks)
1/2 cup of leeks (cut into 3 inch chunks)
1/3 cup of horseradish (drained)
1/3 cup of sour cream

How to Make It:

Put the corned beef into the slow cooker. Rub the seasoning packet onto the top. Add the 3 cups of rutabaga wedges, 2 cups of chopped potatoes, 1 1/2 cups of chunked carrots. Pour the 4 1/2 cups of hot water over the top. Place the cover on the slow cooker and cook on high for 7 1/2 hours. At the last 30 minutes add the 1/2 head of wedged cabbage. While the cabbage is cooking, pull out a cup of the liquid and place in a sauce pan. Turn the heat to high and bring the liquid to a boil. Stir in the 1/3 cup of drained horseradish and the 1/3 cup of sour cream. Pour into a bowl and set aside. Pull the corned beef out to slice. Place the sliced corned beef on a platter. Arrange the vegetables around the corned beef. Add another 1 1/2 cups of the liquid to the horseradish sauce, stir and then pour the over the beef and vegetables and serve.

Makes 6 servings.

Mexican Chicken Fajita Casserole

The delicious fajita seasoning combined with pinto beans and hot diced tomatoes makes this a meal begging for seconds.

What You'll Need:

8 cups of chicken breasts (deboned, skinless, cut into strips, rinsed and dried)
2 cans of pinto beans (16 oz. cans, undrained)
2 cans of tomatoes and peppers (diced 10 oz. cans)
3 tablespoons of canola oil
1 tablespoon of fajita seasoning
salt and pepper

How to Make It:

Pour the 3 tablespoons of canola oil into a skillet and heat to medium high. Rub some salt and pepper into the chicken strips, then cook for 2 minutes each side to sear. Pour the 2 cans of undrained pinto beans into the slow cooker. Place the seared chicken strips on top of the beans. Pour the 2 cans of diced tomatoes and peppers over the chicken. Sprinkle the tablespoon of fajita seasoning over the top. Cover the slow cooker and turn to low and cook for 4 hours.

Makes 4 servings.

Spicy Beef Pot Roast and Noodles

This is a different twist for the pot roast, with some extra spices and served over a bed of hot buttered noodles. This is an all in one meal.

What You'll Need:

1 beef chuck roast (3 pounds)
1 can of tomatoes (crushed, undrained 14.5 oz.)
1 fennel bulb (sliced thin)
2 cups of chicken broth (divided)
2 cups of carrots (chunked)
1/2 cup of onion (sliced thin)
1/3 cup of tomato tapenade (prepared sun-dried)
1/3 cup of parsley (fresh chopped flat leaf)
1/3 cup of flour (all-purpose)
1/4 cup of the juice from fruit cocktail (canned in syrup, divided)
3 tablespoons of canola oil
1 tablespoon of herbes de Provence
2 1/2 teaspoons of garlic (minced)
2 teaspoons of salt + more to taste
1 teaspoon of orange zest (fine grated)
pepper to taste
6 servings of hot cooked egg noodles (buttered)

How to Make It:

First, add 3 tablespoons of canola oil to a skillet and heat to medium high. Rub salt and pepper into the chuck roast and brown in the oil, searing on each side, about 10 minutes each side. Add the 1/3 cup of all-purpose flour in a bowl and whisk in 1 1/2 cups of chicken broth. Pour the can of crushed tomatoes into the slow cooker. Add 3 tablespoons of the fruit cocktail syrup along with the tablespoon of herbes de Provence and the 2 teaspoons of salt and stir. Add the browned chuck roast to the slow cooker. Pour the remaining 1/2 cup of chicken broth to the skillet and stir until it bubbles, then deglaze by scraping with a wooden spoon the meat bits from the pan. Pour this over the meat once it is all scraped up. Add the 1/2 cup of carrots, 1/2 cup of thin sliced onions, sliced fennel, and the 2 1/2 teaspoons of minced garlic over the meat and around it. Carefully pour the flour liquid over the top. Cover and set on high and cook for 4 hours. Then set on low and cook another 2 hours. Remove the meat and chuck up for serving. Place the meat on a serving platter. Add the remaining tablespoon of fruit cocktail syrup along with the 1/3 cup of tomato tapenade, 1/3 cup of chopped fresh flat leaf parsley, and the teaspoon of fine grated orange zest to the liquid in the slow cooker. Dash with salt and pepper. Spoon the vegetables around the meat, and then pour the liquid over the top of the vegetables and meat. Serve over a bed of hot buttered egg noodles.

Macaroni and Cheese Crock

An old time favorite dish cooked up nice, hot, and gooey in the slow cooker.

What You'll Need:

2 1/2 cups of cheddar cheese (sharp grated)
2 cups of macaroni noodles (uncooked)
1 cup of milk
1/2 cup of sour cream
1 can of cheddar cheese soup (condensed 10.75 oz.)
3 eggs (beaten)
4 tablespoons of butter (chopped)
1/2 teaspoon of salt
1/2 teaspoon of dry mustard
1/2 teaspoon of pepper

How to Make It:

First, add a pot of water to the stove and bring to a boil. Add the 2 cups of uncooked macaroni noodles and cook until tender according to package directions. Drain off the water and keep the noodles in the strainer. Turn the slow cooker to low to heat. Add the 4 tablespoons of butter to the pot and stir in the 2 1/2 cups of cheese until the cheese melts. Add the cheese mixture to the slow cooker. In a separate bowl mix the 3 beaten eggs with the cup of milk, 1/2 cup of sour cream, can of condensed cheddar cheese soup, 1/2 teaspoon of salt, 1/2 teaspoon of pepper, and 1/2 teaspoon of dry mustard. Add to the melted cheese and stir. Add the cooked macaroni and toss until all coated. Place lid on slow cooker and cook on low for 3 hours. Stir every half an hour.

Makes 12 servings.

Black Bean Chili

A delicious comfort food is always a hit. Serve it with corn chips or crackers or even a peanut butter sandwich. This is a perfect recipe to use with a beef pot roast you may have previously cooked, just save 1/2 pound for this chili.

What You'll Need:

1/2 pound of beef chuck roast (cooked and cubed)
1 can of crushed tomatoes (28 oz.)
1 can of black beans (drained 15 oz.)
2 cups of water
1/2 cup of onion (diced)
1/4 cup of Monterey jack cheese (shredded)
1 1/2 tablespoons of chili powder
1 tablespoon of garlic (minced)
1 tablespoon of canola oil
salt and pepper

How to Make It:

In a skillet over medium heat, add the tablespoon of canola oil and heat. Stir in the 1/2 cup of diced onion and tablespoon of minced garlic and sauté. Transfer to the slow cooker and add the 1/2 pound of cooked, cubed chuck roast, can of crushed tomatoes, can of black beans, 2 cups of water, 1 1/2 tablespoons of chili powder and dashes of salt and pepper. Cover and heat on low for 2 to 3 hours. Ladle into bowls and garnish with the shredded Monterey jack cheese.

Makes 4 servings.

Beefy Noodles

Enjoy a hot meal in one with just the addition of a side salad and maybe a roll, you will have a perfect beefy meal.

What You'll Need:

2 pounds of stew meat
1 cup of bell peppers (stemmed, seeded, chopped RED)
1/2 cup of onion (sliced)
1/2 cup of beef broth
1/2 cup of sour cream
1/8 cup of dill (fresh chopped)
1/8 cup of parsley (fresh chopped)
2 tablespoons of paprika
2 tablespoons of tomato paste
2 tablespoons of flour (all-purpose)
1 teaspoon of caraway seeds (crushed)
1 teaspoon of garlic (minced)
1 teaspoon of salt
1/4 teaspoon of pepper
8 servings of cooked egg noodles

How to Make It:

Place the 1/2 cup of sliced onions in the bottom of the

slow cooker. In a large zip loc bag add the 2 pounds of stew meat and the 2 tablespoons of all-purpose flour, teaspoon of salt, and 1/4 teaspoon of pepper. Close the bag and shake, evenly coat each piece of beef. Add the coated beef on top of the onions. Add the 1 cup of red bell peppers and sprinkle with the teaspoon of minced garlic. In a bowl, add the 1/2 cup of beef broth, 2 tablespoons of paprika, 2 tablespoons of tomato paste, and teaspoon of crushed caraway seeds and stir. Pour over the beef. Add the cover to the slow cooker and cook on high for 4 hours or on low for 8 hours. When done, remove the lid and turn off. Let it stand for 10 minutes. Stir in the 1/2 cup of sour cream along with the 1/8 cups of fresh chopped dill and parsley. Salt and pepper to taste. Spoon over a bed of fresh hot egg noodles.

Makes 8 servings.

Shredded Turkey Sandwiches

Whoever loves a good turkey will love this recipe that creates a tender and juicy shredded turkey sandwich with a nice serving of slaw or even delicious over a salad.

What You'll Need:

4 turkey thighs
1/2 cup of onion (chopped)
1/2 cup of ketchup
1/4 cup of brown sugar (light and packed)
2 tablespoons of yellow mustard
1 tablespoon of apple cider vinegar
1 tablespoon of chili powder
1 teaspoon of cumin (ground)
1 teaspoon of salt
1/2 teaspoon of pepper

How to Make It:

Place the 1/2 cup of chopped onion on the bottom of the slow cooker. Remove the skin from the turkey thighs. Mix the tablespoon of chili powder, teaspoon of ground cumin, teaspoon of salt and the 1/2 teaspoon of pepper. Then rub the seasoning on the turkey thighs. Place the thighs on the onions in the slow cooker. Mix the 1/2 cup of ketchup with the 2 tablespoons of yellow mustard and stir in the tablespoon of apple cider vinegar. Pour over the turkey thighs. Place the lid on the slow cooker and cook for 6 hours on low or 3 hours on high. Once done, remove the lid, turn off slow cooker and let sit for 10 minutes. Pull out the turkey thighs and "pull" or "shred" the meat from the bones. Discard the bones. Serve on buns or bread or over a salad.

Makes 6 servings.

Round Steak

A delicious round steak that goes well with steamed vegetables and a salad.

What You'll Need:

1 1/2 pounds of round steak (cut into bite-sized strips)
1 can of tomatoes (diced 14.5 oz.)
1 can of water (using the tomatoes can)
1/2 cup of onions (strips)
1/2 cup of bell peppers (strips)
1 teaspoon of garlic powder
1 teaspoon of garlic (minced)
salt and pepper
flour (all-purpose)
canola oil

How to Make It:

Rub salt, pepper and the teaspoon of garlic powder onto the round stead strips. Roll the strips in some all-purpose flour. Pour some canola oil in a skillet and turn heat to medium high. Cook the round steak until brown on all sides. Add the meat to the slow cooker. In a bowl, mix the can of tomatoes, can of water with the 1/2 cup of onion strips, 1/2 cup of bell pepper strips, and the teaspoon of minced garlic. Pour over the round steak. Place a lid on the slow cooker and cook on low for 90 minutes. Check to make sure the meat stays covered with liquid. Continue to cook until the steak is cooked to your desired done, as well done, medium, or rare.

Makes 4 servings.

Shrimp Creole Casserole

For those who love to partake in the seafood with a New Orleans flare, you will love this shrimp Creole made from the slow cooker.

What You'll Need:

1.5 pounds of shrimp (peeled and deveined)
1 can of tomatoes (14 oz., diced)
1 can of tomato sauce (8 oz.)
1/2 cup of bell peppers (green diced)
1/2 cup of onions (diced)
1/2 cup of celery (diced)
2 tablespoons of olive oil
1 tablespoon of hot sauce
1 tablespoon of Worcestershire sauce
1 teaspoon of sugar (granulated)
1 teaspoon of chili powder
salt and pepper
cooked rice
green onions (for garnishment)

How to Make It:

First, heat the 2 tablespoons of olive oil in a skillet on medium high. Add the 1/2 cups of diced green bell peppers, onions, and celery and sauté. Stir in the teaspoon of chili powder. Transfer to the slow cooker. Add the can of tomatoes, can of tomato sauce, tablespoon of hot sauce, tablespoon of Worcestershire sauce, teaspoon of granulated sugar, and salt and pepper to taste. Cover and cook on high for three hours. Add the 1.5 pounds of shrimp and cook for 3 more minutes. Turn off heat and transfer to a large serving bowl. Serve over cooked rice and garnish with the green onions.

Makes 8 servings.

Jamaica Chicken

Enjoy the flavor of the Caribbean in this delicious one dish meal with chicken and all of the favorite Jamaican flavors.

What You'll Need:

4 pounds of chicken thighs (skinless)
1 can of tomato sauce (15 oz.)
1 can of coconut milk (14 oz.)
1 can of red beans (15 oz., drained)
1 avocado (diced)
2 cups of white rice (instant)
1 cup of water
1 cup of onions (sliced)
1 cup of celery (chopped)
1 cup of carrots (chopped)
1/4 cup of lime juice
1/4 cup of cilantro leaves (fresh chopped)
1/4 cup of scallions (chopped)
1 tablespoon of chipotle chilies (+1 teaspoon, minced in adobo sauce)
1 teaspoon of garlic (minced)
1 teaspoon of thyme (dried)
1/2 teaspoon of lime zest (fine grate)
salt and pepper
lime wedges (garnishment)

How to Make It:

Place the cups of sliced onions, chopped celery, and chopped carrots in the bottom of the slow cooker. Sprinkle salt and pepper on the chicken thighs and place the thighs on top of the vegetables. In a bowl, combine the can of tomato sauce with the 1/4 cup of lime juice, tablespoon and teaspoon of chipotle chilies, with the teaspoon of minced garlic. Stir and pour over the chicken and vegetables. Cover the slow cooker and cook on high for 4 hours or low for 8 hours. Right before serving add the 2 cups of instant white rice, cans of coconut milk, drained red beans, teaspoon of dried thyme, and the 1/2 teaspoon of fine grated lime zest in a sauce pan. Turn to high and just before boiling, turn to low to simmer. Cover and simmer for five minutes. Toss in the 1/4 cup of chopped scallions and season with salt and pepper. Serve the chicken and vegetables over a bed of the rice.

Makes 4 servings.

Jambalaya

Here is a Cajun favorite dish made with both chicken and shrimp.

What You'll Need:

1 pound of chicken breasts (boneless, skinless cut into chunks)
1 pound of shrimp (peeled, deveined)
1/2 pound of hot turkey sausage (diced)
1 can of tomatoes (28 oz. diced)
2 cups of rice (cooked)
1 cup of chicken broth
1/2 cup of onions (chopped)
1/2 cup of bell pepper (green, seeded, chopped)
1/2 cup of celery (chopped)
2 bay leaves
2 teaspoons of oregano (dried)
2 teaspoons of Cajun seasoning
1 teaspoon of hot sauce
1/2 teaspoon of dried thyme

How to Make It:

Add the pound of chunked chicken breasts, 1/2 pound of hot turkey sausage (diced), can of diced tomatoes, cup of chicken broth, 1/2 cup of chopped onion, 1/2 cup of chopped green bell pepper, and the 1/2 cup of chopped celery into the slow cooker. In a small bowl combine the 2 teaspoons of dried oregano, 2 teaspoons of Cajun seasoning, teaspoon of hot sauce, and the 1/2 teaspoon of dried thyme. Add to the chicken and vegetables. Add the 2 bay leaves. Cover and cook on high for 3 hours or low for 6 to 7 hours. At the last five minutes, add the pound of peeled deveined shrimp and cook. Remove the bay leaves. Serve over a bed of rice.

Makes 4 servings.

Spicy Black-Eyed Peas

A delicious main dish which will go perfect with a pan of hot corn bread and a salad. There's enough here to have for leftovers.

What You'll Need:

4 cans of black-eyed peas (drained and rinsed - 14 oz. each)
1 can of tomatoes and chili peppers (14.5 oz., drained)
1 1/2 cups of bell pepper (green chopped)
1 cup of onion (chopped)
1 cup of turkey ham (diced)
1/4 cup of butter
1 tablespoon of seasoned salt
1 teaspoon of garlic (minced)

How to Make It:

Stir together the 4 cans of black-eyed peas, 1 can of tomatoes and chili peppers,)
1 1/2 cups of bell pepper, 1 cup of onion, 1 cup of turkey ham, 1/4 cup of butter, 1 tablespoon of seasoned salt, and 1 teaspoon of garlic in the slow cooker. Place on the lid and cook on low setting for four hours.

Makes 12 servings.

Beef Pepper Steak

A delicious way to serve steak that is fall off the fork tender and tasty.   Delicious over rice.

What You'll Need:

2 pounds of beef sirloin (cut into small strips)
1 can of tomatoes (stewed, undrained)
1 beef bouillon cube
2 cups of bell peppers (red, cut into strips)
1/2 cup of onions (chopped)
1/4 cup of water (hot)
3 tablespoons of soy sauce
3 tablespoons of canola oil
1 tablespoon of cornstarch
1 teaspoon of sugar (granulated)
1 teaspoon of salt
garlic powder
cooked rice for 6 servings

How to Make It:

Sprinkle the garlic powder over the beef sirloin strips. Add the 3 tablespoons of canola oil to a skillet to brown the beef sirloin strips. Add the browned strips to the slow cooker. In a small bowl or cup mix the 1/4 cup of hot water with the beef bouillon cube to dissolve it completely. Stir in the tablespoon of cornstarch. Pour the liquid over the beef strips. Add the can of undrained stewed tomatoes, 2 cups of red bell pepper strips, and the 1/2 cup of chopped onion. In a cup mix the 3 tablespoons of soy sauce with the teaspoon of sugar and salt. Pour over the contents of the slow cooker. Cover and cook on low for 8 hours or high for 4 hours. Serve over a bed of cooked rice.

Makes 6 servings.

Vegetarian Chili

For those of you who are on a meat free diet or who are just trying to avoid extra meat, try this very delicious all vegetable chili.

What You'll Need:

1 can of black bean soup (19 oz. can)
1 can of vegetarian baked beans (16 oz.)
1 can of kidney beans (15 oz., drained and rinsed)
1 can of corn (whole kernel, drained 15 oz.)
1 can of tomatoes (chopped and pureed 14.5 oz.)
1 cup of celery (chopped)
1/2 cup of onions (chopped)
1/2 cup of bell peppers (green, chopped)
1 tablespoon of parsley (dried)
1 tablespoon of oregano (dried)
1 tablespoon of basil (dried)
1 tablespoon of chili powder
1 teaspoon of garlic (minced)

How to Make It:

Add the 1 can of black bean soup, 1 can of vegetarian baked beans, 1 can of kidney beans, 1 can of corn, 1 can of tomatoes, 1 cup of celery, 1/2 cup of onions,

1/2 cup of bell peppers, 1 tablespoon of parsley, 1 tablespoon of oregano, 1 tablespoon of basil, 1 tablespoon of chili powder, and 1 teaspoon of garlic into the slow cooker and stir. Cover and cook on high for 2 hours.

Makes 8 servings.

Chicken and Dumplings

This is an all-time favorite for many. Nothing fills the tummy and warms the heart like a delicious bowl of chicken and dumplings.

What You'll Need:

4 chicken breast halves (boneless, skinless)
2 cans of biscuits (refrigerator, 10 oz. each torn into bite-sized pieces)
1 "family sized" can of cream of chicken soup (condensed)
1/2 cup of onion (diced)
2 tablespoons of butter
chicken broth
salt and pepper

How to Make It:

Add the 4 chicken breast halves, 1/2 cup of onion, and the 2 tablespoons of butter into the slow cooker. In a bowl, whisk together at least a cup of chicken broth with the family sized can of condensed cream of chicken soup. Pour over the chicken. Salt and pepper and stir. Add more chicken broth until all the chicken is completely covered with liquid. Cover with a lid and cook on high for 5 hours and 30 minutes. Remove the chicken and "pull" apart by shredding with a fork. Replace the chicken and add the bite sized raw biscuit pieces and cook for another half an hour. Salt and pepper to taste. Enjoy.

Serving suggestion, add a can of English peas (drained) during the last half hour for added color and flavor.

Makes 8 servings.

French Dip Au Jus

This makes the most tender beef sandwiches and a savory au jus sauce for dipping.

What You'll Need:

4 pounds of rump roast
8 French rolls
1 can of French onion soup (condensed, 10.5 oz.)
1 1/2 cups of beef broth
1 1/2 cups of ginger ale
2 tablespoons of butter

How to Make It:

Remove as much fat from the rump roast before placing in the slow cooker. In a bowl, mix the can of condensed French onion soup with the 1 1/2 cups of beef broth, 1 1/2 cups of ginger ale with a whisk. Pour over the rump roast. Cover and cook on low for 7 hours. Preheat the oven to 350 degrees Fahrenheit, once the meat is cooked, slice the 8 French rolls in half lengthwise (if not already sliced). Spread butter on them and bake in the oven for ten minutes. Remove the roast and slice thin. Place on the rolls as sandwiches. Serve with a bowl of ladled meat liquid or "au jus" for dipping.

Makes 8 servings.

Chicken Stroganoff

This stroganoff is tasty made with chicken breasts and cream cheese. This is a "can't go wrong" recipe.

What You'll Need:

4 chicken breast halves (skinless and boneless)
1 package of cream cheese (8 oz. package)
1 can of cream of chicken soup (10.75 condensed)
1 packet of Italian salad dressing mix (dry)
2 tablespoons of butter
cooked egg noodles for 4 servings

How to Make It:

Place the chicken breast halves in the bottom of the slow cooker. Cut the 2 tablespoons of butter into bits and sprinkle over the chicken. Sprinkle the packet of Italian dressing mix over the butter and chicken. Cover and cook on low for 5 and a half hours. Add the package of cream cheese and the can of condensed cream of chicken soup and cook for 30 more minutes. Serve over cooked egg noodles.

Makes 4 servings.

Spaghetti

This spaghetti is so good you will have people asking you to make it over and over. The recipe makes enough for leftovers or to freeze.

What You'll Need:

1 can of tomatoes (28 oz., crushed)
1 can of tomatoes (28 oz., diced)
1 can of tomato sauce (10 oz.)
1 can of tomato paste (6 oz.)
1/2 pound of turkey kielbasa (chopped)
1/2 pound of ground beef (extra lean)
1/2 pound of ground turkey breast
6 squash (yellow, diced)
5 bay leaves
1 1/2 cups of onions (chopped)
1/2 cup of bell peppers (green minced)
1/4 cup of olive oil (extra virgin)
2 teaspoons of thyme (dried)
1 1/2 teaspoons of garlic (minced)
1 1/2 teaspoons of basil (dried)
1 teaspoon of marjoram (dried)
1 teaspoon of black pepper
1/2 teaspoon of oregano (dried)
Cooked spaghetti noodles (enough to handle up to 12

servings)

How to Make It:

Add the cans of crushed tomatoes, diced tomatoes, tomato sauce and tomato paste to the slow cooker and stir to combine. Add the 1/2 pound of chopped turkey kielbasa. Cover and turn to high. Add the 1/4 cup of extra virgin olive oil to a skillet and heat to medium. Add the 6 diced squash, 1 1/2 cups of chopped onions, 1/2 cup of minced green bell peppers, and the 1 1/2 teaspoons of minced garlic and sauté. Add the sautéed vegetables to the tomato mixture in the slow cooker. Add the 1/2 pounds of extra lean ground beef and the ground turkey breast into the skillet. Turn to medium high and brown the meat. Drain the grease and with a fork crumble it to fine bits. Add into the slow cooker and stir. Sprinkle the 2 teaspoons of dried thyme, 1 1/2 teaspoons of dried basil, 1 teaspoon of dried marjoram, teaspoon of black pepper, and the 1/2 teaspoon of dried oregano into the spaghetti sauce. Add the 5 bay leaves. Cover and cook for 2 hours on high. Remove the cover and cook for an additional hour. Serve over a bed of spaghetti noodles.

Makes 12 servings.

5 Day Meal Plan -

Each meal can be improvised by adding extra bread or rolls, or steamed vegetables, a salad, or whatever you feel is appropriate. For breakfasts you may want to add toast or biscuits and depending on which recipe you may want to add some protein like turkey sausage or a glass of milk. The lunches are soups, stews and macaroni and cheese. These are fine by themselves, but you can add crackers or bread with them. Enjoy!

Day 1 –

Breakfast - Cranberry Oatmeal
Snack - piece of fruit
Lunch - Chicken Noodle Cream Soup
Snack - hummus and pita chips
Supper - Mexican Chicken Fajita Casserole
Dessert - Quick Tapioca Pudding

Day 2 –

Breakfast - Raspberry Coconut Rice Pudding
Snack - trail mix
Lunch - Macaroni and Cheese Crock
Snack - piece of fruit

Supper - Spicy Beef Pot Roast and Noodles
Dessert - Quick Chocolate Nut Clusters

Day 3 –

Breakfast - Turkey Bacon and Egg Casserole
Snack - piece of fruit
Lunch - French Onion Soup
Snack - trail mix
Supper - Spicy Black-eyed Peas
Dessert - Chocolate Mocha Bread Pudding

Day 4 –

Breakfast - Breakfast Cheese Strata with Vegetables
Snack - nuts
Lunch - Split Pea Soup
Snack - piece of fruit
Supper - Round Steak
Dessert - Carrot Cake

Day 5 –

Breakfast - Cherry Croissant Pudding
Snack - piece of fruit
Lunch - Mexican Tortilla Soup
Snack - nuts

Supper - Black Bean Chili
Dessert - Peach Cheesecake

Conclusion

We hope you enjoyed browsing through the slow cooker recipes and hope you have tried a few. Many will become favorites, so be prepared!

It is okay to adapt these recipes and substitute ingredients if you wish. You can add to or take away from, but if you do there is no guarantee it will be as good as the original recipe. But you never know until you try it. You may come up with a new food masterpiece.

Take care of your slow cooker. Clean it well after each use, not just the food container, but the outer body and the cord. Remember you cannot submerse the outer body or the cords in water, so use caution when cleaning. A damp cloth and some elbow grease will go a long ways in making the outside look nice.

CPSIA information can be obtained
at www.ICGtesting.com
Printed in the USA
LVOW10s0810141217
559689LV00018B/781/P